OUT

OF

THE

WOODS

Dear children and adults who are reading this book, I think all children's dreams should come true, and this has been my dream for many years to have my own book, and here it is – you've either started or finished reading it . . .

Whoever you are and wherever you are, I hope you're spandandall*.

Betsy

*Spandandall: feeling good, upbeat and excited all at the same time.

OUT
OF
THE
WOODS

A tale of positivity, kindness and courage

BETSY GRIFFIN

With Sue Belfrage

Illustrated by Emanuel Santos

Foreword

Every now and then a very special book comes along that has the power to help people in many ways. Luckily for you, this is one of those very books. Betsy, as you'll know, is also very special. And if you don't know, you're about to find out.

My name is Fearne Cotton and I'm a broadcaster – which means I talk on the TV and radio – and an author. Let me tell you how I know Betsy, and why I know you'll love this book.

I first found out about Betsy because she is the daughter of the cousin of one of my best, and oldest friends. On many occasions I had heard from my friend Becky about how brilliant Betsy was, but it wasn't until I watched Betsy's YouTube channel that I truly understood what a wise, amazing, and impactful person she is.

I was instantly struck by Betsy's calm, confident delivery, and really pulled in by her charm, wit, and wisdom. I have learned so many lessons from watching her videos. Not only are they uplifting, they are also jam-packed with anecdotal advice for life.

Betsy is also unstoppable. One of my favourite videos from her channel features her talking cheerfully, just after waking up from an operation. She asked her mum and dad if she could film some of her thoughts straight after her operation, and once again, she calmly put her own life experience out there for us to learn from. She also showed us her favourite cuddly tiger – which is ginormous.

From advice on meditation, to how to view the world with a more positive attitude, Betsy has a lot to say. I love hearing her talk and crack jokes, and also use her favourite word – 'spandandall'!

Like many others out there, I've not only taken heed of Betsy's advice, but have also been deeply moved by her story and determination. She has dealt with multiple medical procedures and healthcare issues from a young age. She is blind, but never lets any adverse situations get in the way of her messages. Betsy is a true example of strength and positivity, which are two attributes I think many of us would like to have. By listening to other's stories, we can become stronger and more positive in our general outlook.

Each time I watch one of Betsy's videos I feel truly boosted and ready to face new challenges.

This book promises to do the same. Its rich stories and vivid descriptions will give you a beautiful dose of escapism and enjoyment, as well as teach you some of the incredible life lessons that Betsy has to offer. Do you like adventures? I do! Betsy has many for us to go on, so get ready to have some fun and soak up some wisdom along the way.

Fearne Cotton

CONTENTS

Betsy's Story

As soon as you meet Betsy Griffin you discover that she is somebody very special. Should you be invited to her home for tea and cake, the chances are you will be greeted with a big smile and a warm hug. There is bound to be music, singing, dancing and laughter. Once you have chatted to her parents, Stuart and Rochelle, and her younger sisters, Ava and Faith, Betsy may offer to take you by the hand and give you a guided tour of her room, where she will introduce you to her collection of favourite furry animals. The most special of these is Jess, the toy dog given to Betsy when she was little more than a baby and undergoing a gruelling eighteen-month course of intensive chemotherapy.

In 2016, when Betsy was only two years old, her family learned that she had a rare form of large and inoperable brain tumour. It was causing irreparable damage to her optic nerve. The chemo did little to shrink the tumour yet Betsy endured the treatment's side-effects and complications with courage and positivity. By now registered blind, she won the hearts of every doctor and nurse who cared for her, and, as is Betsy's way, proved to be as curious and interested in their lives as she was determined to enjoy every single moment of her own. Although her tumour initially stabilised when she was placed on a breakthrough drugs trial, she has had to endure many more hospital visits, major operations and procedures over the years. She still lives under the shadow of the tumour's return and continues to take regular medication.

Throughout it all, Betsy has determinedly tackled every challenge she has faced. She joined a mainstream school, learned Braille on her very own Brailler, and enjoys learning the piano and creating her own songs. Today, she enjoys art (although she finds it hard to make out shapes and colours with her impaired vision) and can even dart around on her sister Ava's scooter.

When Covid-19 struck fear across nations, Betsy announced at the age of six that she wanted to 'spread inspiration around the world, like you spread Nutella on bread'. With the encouragement and support of her family and friends, she launched Betsy's Positive Videos, her own YouTube channel, to raise money for charities who help children with life limiting or terminal illnesses dreams come true. Her videos feature inspiring conversations about everything from creativity and gratitude to resilience and the power of kindness.

While young in years, Betsy is what you might call an old soul. She admits there are times when she finds things difficult, but she is determined not to let these get the better of her and chooses to focus on how lucky she is. When she performed as a soloist on British television in a concert led by choirmaster and broadcaster Gareth Malone, he remarked that she'd been through a lot for a little girl. With a shrug and a thoughtful smile, Betsy replied, 'Well, that's life, Gareth.'

As you will discover, Betsy is a natural storyteller. In this deceptively simple fable, she shares insights and wisdom that can help us all, whatever our age, encouraging us to open our hearts, learn, love and follow our truth, no matter what may stand in our path.

Watch Betsy's Positive Videos on YouTube here
www.youtube.com/channel/UCfmZ0v3rV79E3Qf8bhXrBKQ

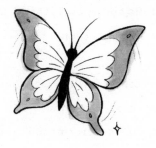

CHAPTER 1

Here and Now

There was no wind.

A hint of fresh grass hung in the air, scenting the Meadowlands with a gentle summer perfume.

A brief rustle. The shuffling of feet.

Branches snapped, cracking like whips.

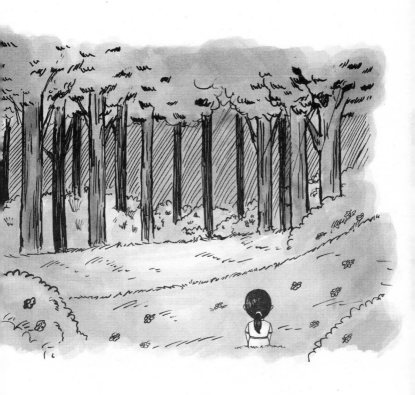

Something moved.

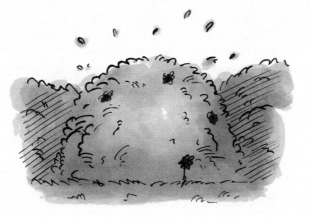

Betsy listened.

Leaves fluttered and whispered. But this was something else. Something bigger.

The patter of running feet?

A creature dashed into the woods, disturbing the peace at the edge of the meadow.

Footsteps light, quick, and darting. An animal scurried, fast, panicked

. . . afraid.

Betsy heard it scramble through the undergrowth, coming closer, towards a thicket near her feet.

She crouched down and listened again.

A low murmur sounded from behind the leaves. Something hurt, or maybe lost?

A faint whimper reached her ears.

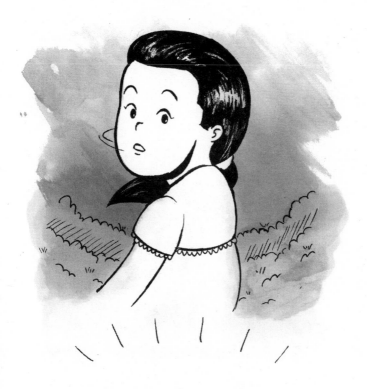

Betsy turned to her sisters,
Ava and baby Faith.

'Listen,' Betsy said. 'Can you hear that?'

'Hear what?' Ava could only hear Faith giggling at something on the ground.

'It sounds like an animal crying.'

Ava looked around. 'I can't see anything.'

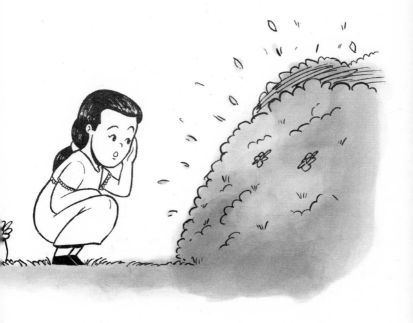

Betsy thought for a second, then made a decision.

'Stay here with Faith; I'm going to investigate.
If I'm not back soon, fetch help.'

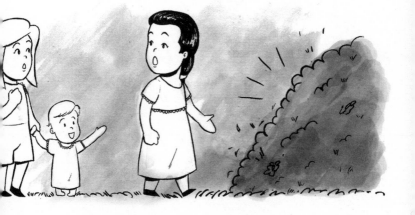

And without hesitating, Betsy wriggled into the dense bushes and disappeared from view.

She picked her way under brambles that snagged her thin cotton dress, keeping her head low.

Scratchy twigs grazed her bare arms and legs.

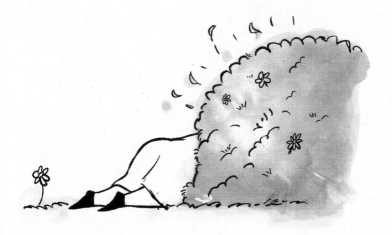

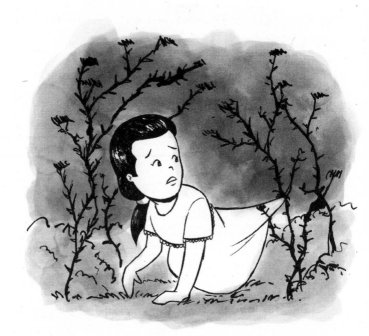

The air turned dank and cold. The heat of the sun couldn't reach through the foliage.

Goosebumps chilled her skin. Betsy heard the short, panting breath of another living creature.

She felt more space around her and stood up.

No branches grabbed at her clothes, although she could still smell trees nearby and the scent of damp soil.

She stumbled forwards, her feet sliding over the slippery, stony surface.

Was she in

a tunnel?

Or was it

a cave?

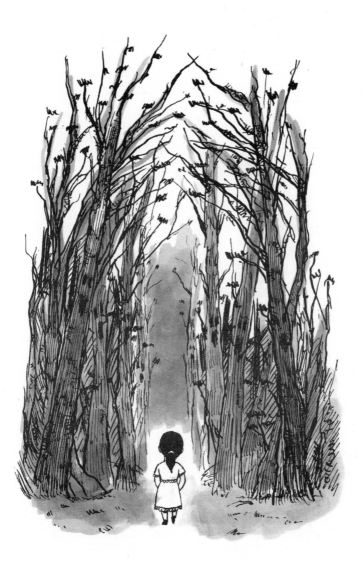

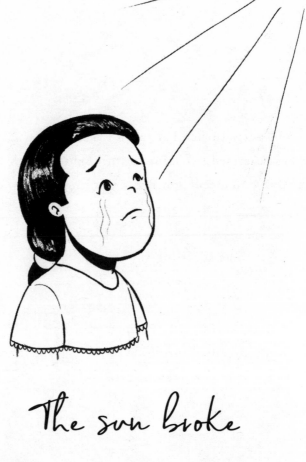

The sun broke
through the clouds

and Betsy turned her face to the sky as a welcome
heat caressed her skin, and brought warmth to her
body. Pine needles and mulch squelched underfoot.
A tang filled her nostrils.

The scuffling sounds of tiny claws
moved in her direction.

Betsy stood still. Then something small and
soft bundled into her legs. She gasped, then
reached down.

Her fingers sank into a fuzzy bundle of thick and luxurious fur.

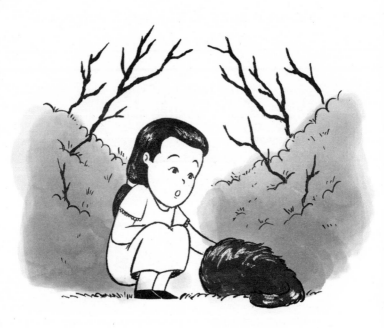

Small, wet licks tickled her hand. Yelps of relief.
A cold, wet nose. The milky scent of a puppy.

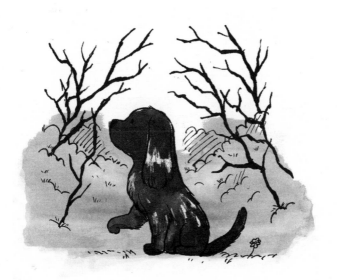

Betsy felt the urge to hold it tight and snuggle close.

She put out her arms and a furry little body
hurled itself into them.

Betsy pressed her face into the puppy's side.
Its fur was warm and soft, but tangled with
knots of mud.

She breathed the cosy, homely smell of biscuits,
cinnamon, and newly cut hay, mingled with hints
of dirt. But not the rich, earthy scent of the forest.
Instead, Betsy sensed the sickly sweet smell of a
terrified and lost animal.

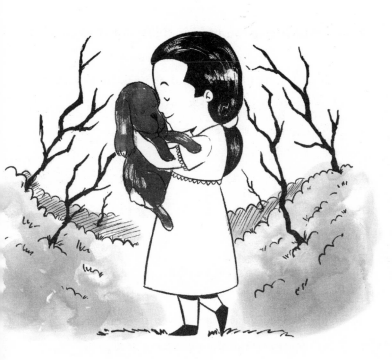

She felt round its neck. No collar.
Perhaps it had fallen off.

'What shall I call you?' Betsy stroked the puppy's
soft head soothingly.

A hint of
orange zest
reached her nose.

'How about Clementine?'

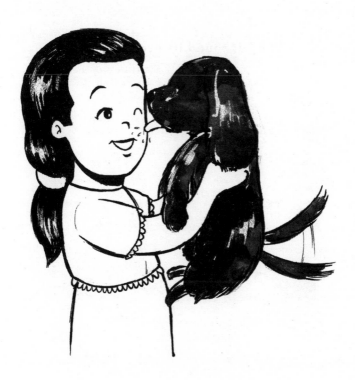

The puppy licked her chin. That had to be a yes.

'I need to make you a lead of some sort if I'm going to get you home,' Betsy told the puppy. 'So we don't lose each other.'

She thought for a moment, then she extended her arm as far as it would go.

Long strands of ivy and thick honeysuckle vines dangled from the surrounding trees, and skimmed her outstretched hands.

She grabbed hold and tugged hard, thinking about how she and Ava sometimes plaited each other's hair.

A strong tendril of ivy came loose.

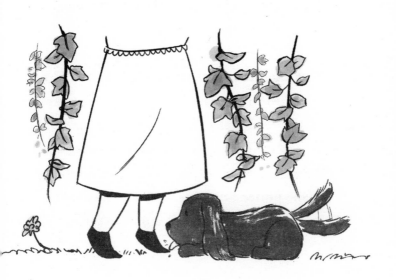

With the puppy curled up safely at her feet, Betsy worked furiously and quickly as she wove a makeshift lead, her hands moving over and under each other in a well-rehearsed pattern.

She pulled at each end of her creation.
It stayed firm and didn't break.

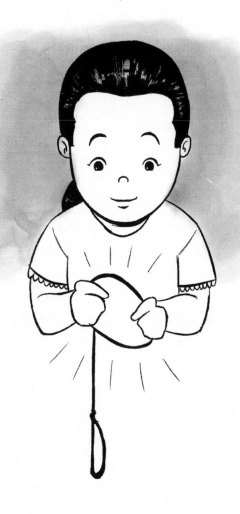

'That should do it!' She smiled happily to herself.

She paused.

The tunnel was the way she had come.

But where was it?

Her fingers reached down and stroked the puppy,
which sat like a heavy bag of flour, weighing
down her feet.

Clementine was no longer shaking. Instead, she snuffled gently at Betsy's fingers, as Betsy tied the lead slowly around the puppy's neck.

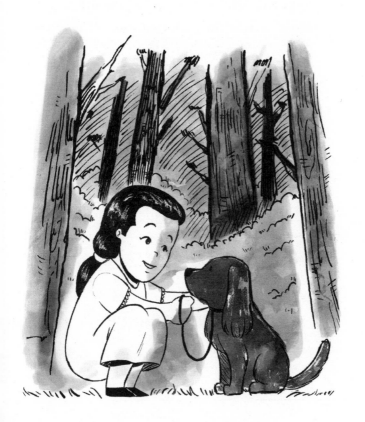

'Let's go home,' she said. They headed off together, Betsy confidently leading the way, but after a while, Betsy stopped.

nothing seemed quite right.

The smells were different and the ground beneath her feet didn't feel familiar.

'Oh dear!' Betsy sighed. 'Perhaps this isn't the right way after all.'

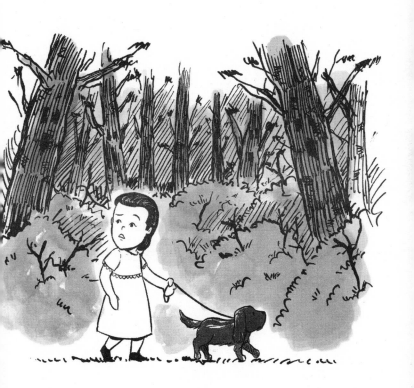

'Can I help?'

A voice as clear as a silver bell tinkled in Betsy's ear.

She swung round in the speaker's direction.
Floating on the light wind, something hovered
close to her nose.

Its wings flickered in the breeze, as it fluttered on an upward gust of wind.

Betsy lifted her head in its direction, sensing a puff of air as gentle wings silently fanned her face. A butterfly.

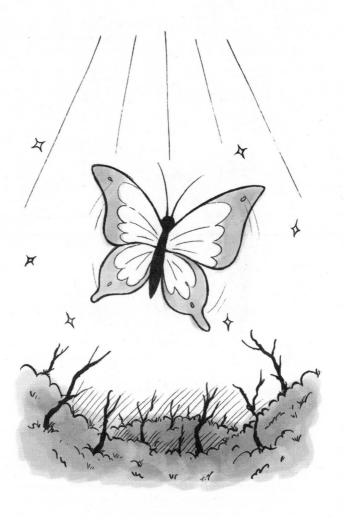

'Thank you, but I don't think you can help.'
Betsy shrugged apologetically. 'You're even
smaller than me.'

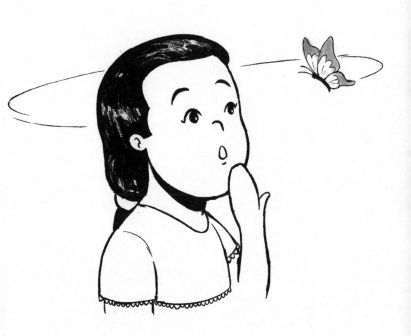

The butterfly sniffed.

'I may be small,
but inside
I'm a giant.

I might just surprise you.'

Betsy chuckled and Clementine yipped. 'I'm trying to get this puppy and me home safely,' said Betsy. 'Do you know where we are?'

'You are here,' said the butterfly.

'Yes, I realize that, but I'm not sure which way to go from here.' Betsy turned in a slow circle. 'There seem to be so many directions to choose from.'

'Ah, in that case,

let your mind
show you
the way.'

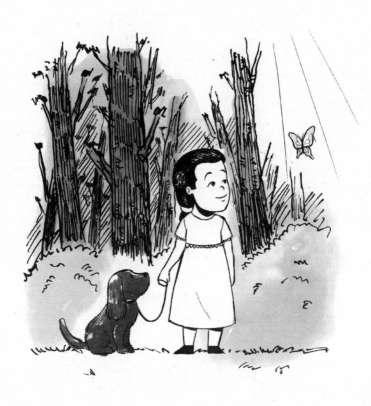

The butterfly stroked Betsy's nose with its wings.

The sensation was instantly relaxing. Her mind cleared. 'How do I do that?'

'You don't need to do anything,' the butterfly said.

'Just be in the moment and let your mind do the rest.'

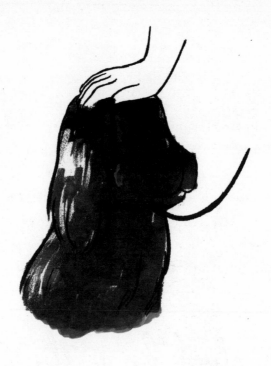

Clementine's damp nose nuzzled at Betsy's hand,
as Betsy stroked the puppy's soft, fluffy head.

'We can't just sit here and wait, when there is
far to go,' she thought aloud. 'But what if we
get even more lost?'

The butterfly landed gently on Betsy's fingers.

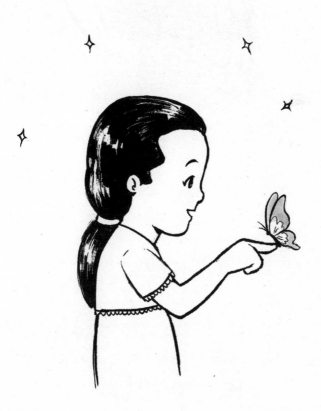

'Can you control the future?'

it asked with a flutter.

'no.'

'Can you change the past?'

'no.'

'Then stop worrying
about the future
and the past,'

the butterfly suggested. 'Enjoy this moment of
sunshine. Sit back, close your eyes and breathe
deeply. Let the warmth caress your face.
Let your thoughts drift like an early summer
morning, when the dew washes everything clean.'

'But what do I do if I can't stop worrying about
getting home?'

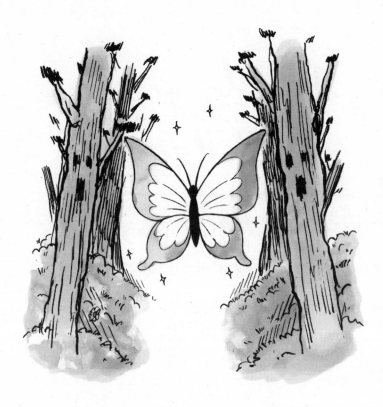

'If you have an
annoying thought,
shoo it away
and let it go.'

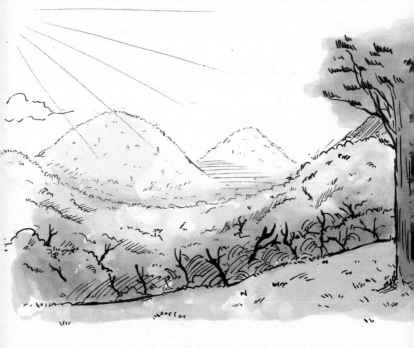

The butterfly fluttered into the air.

'And if I do that, then what will happen?'
asked Betsy.

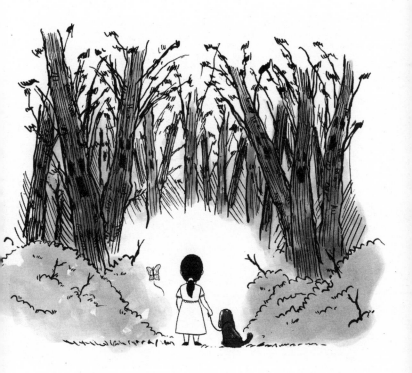

'Nothing will happen!' The butterfly hovered close to Betsy's ear, then whispered, 'That's the point.'

Betsy took a step forward and stubbed her toe on a fallen log. She sat down and drew the puppy onto her lap.

Clementine wriggled, but then relaxed. Soon gentle snores came from her little mouth as her chest rose and fell in a heavy doze. Betsy's thoughts buzzed around her mind like bees busying about a garden. She closed her eyes and pushed away her troublesome thoughts.

She didn't need to worry, she told herself.

Not anymore.

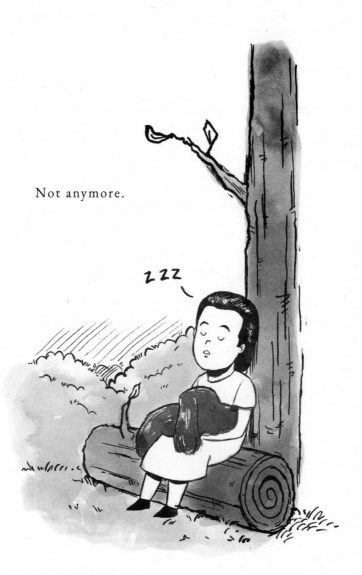

But could she really do that? In her mind

she imagined

sweeping niggling

doubts out of

her head with a

large broom.

Pushing any negative thoughts out through her ears and nose like clouds of dust, she chuckled.

The fluttering of the butterfly brought her back to the present. Its delicate wings tickled her cheeks like farewell kisses.

Betsy opened her eyes. Clementine had grown heavy in her arms. Her paws twitched, as if she was running in her dreams.

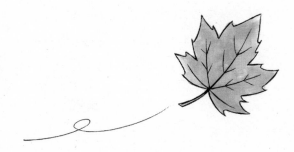

Betsy called out to the butterfly, but there was no
reply. The insect had flown off.

Betsy felt a lightness in her chest and knew without
any doubt that she had an inner map all of her own –
one that would help her find the right way home.

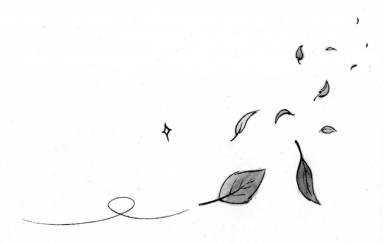

Whatever lay ahead
no longer seemed
so frightening.

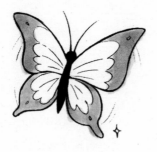

CHAPTER 2

*Spandandall!**

*Spandandall: feeling good, upbeat and
excited all at the same time.

Clementine sniffed the way ahead as she and Betsy negotiated a twisting path through the densely packed trees. Betsy wondered if the puppy might pick up a familiar scent that would lead them in the right direction. Where were they going?

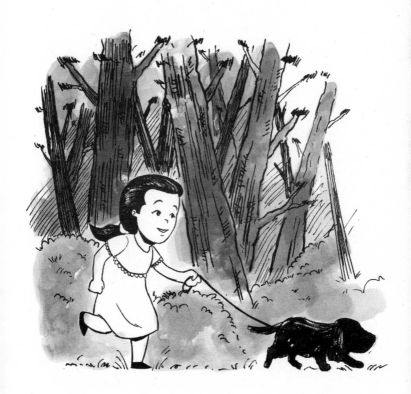

After a while, the ground became less springy underfoot. They had reached a clearing.

Long grass, dry to the touch, tickled Betsy's ankles and legs. She ran her hands over it.

Wild flowers powdered Betsy's palms with sticky pollen.

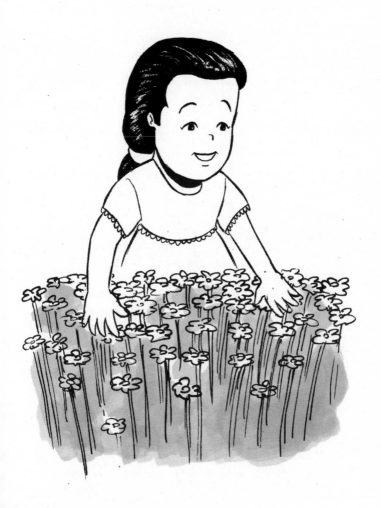

Betsy breathed in its intoxicating scent.

The sultry sun beat down, its hot rays soothing her eyelids.

Clementine started to yip as a large animal
thundered past.

'What was that?' asked Betsy.

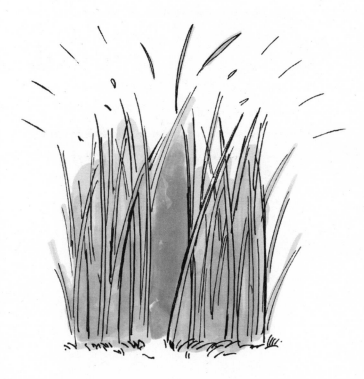

'I beg your pudding!' a breathless voice
gasped from somewhere in the grass.
'I think you mean who, not what!'

'Sorry.' Betsy tried again. 'May I ask who you are?'

She reached forward and her fingers brushed
the velvety tips of two long ears poking out of
the dry grass.

Her feet felt the vibrations as the animal thumped past her, and jumped up and down.

Clementine pulled at her lead excitedly, but didn't seem to be scared.

The bouncing sensation stopped. 'You're too big to be a rabbit,' Betsy decided.

'I'm a happy hare,' laughed the voice.

'And whenever
I'm happy –'

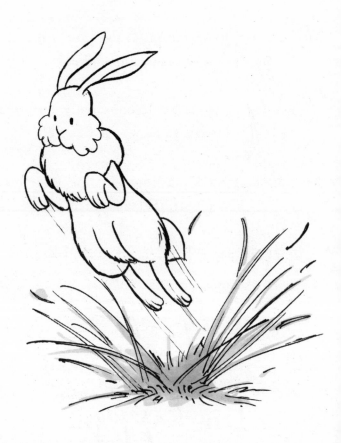

the hare caught her breath

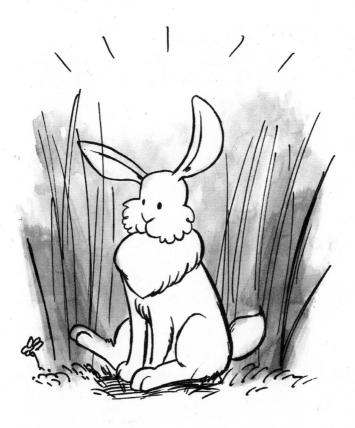

'–I get into a state
I call spandandall,
which is a word
I invented.

It makes me want to leap about. You should try it.'

Betsy pondered briefly. 'At the moment, I'm not sure Clementine and I have very much to feel happy about. We're trying to get back home to the Meadowlands, but I suspect we're walking in circles.'

The hare moved closer, until Betsy sensed its
thrumming footsteps stop right in front of her.

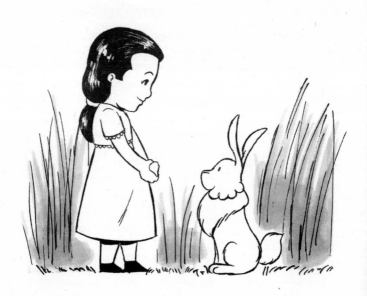

Clementine calmed down, no longer pulling on her lead, and sniffed curiously at the hare's fluffy tail.

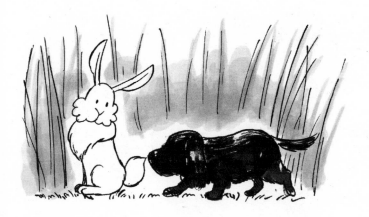

'There is always something to feel happy about.'

The hare rubbed its ears with a paw.
'Today, I'm happy because,

as soon as I woke
up, I thought
of at least three
things that I am
grateful for:

a tasty plant I nibbled yesterday;

lots of space in which to race about;

and the company of all my family and friends
in the woods.'

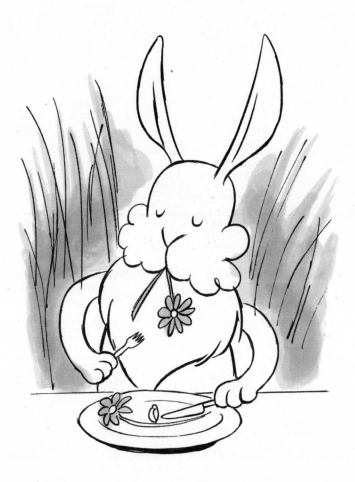

Betsy's chest tightened and her whole body ached when the hare mentioned its family.

'Poor Clementine's family must be missing her horribly. And mine must be worried too. I asked my sisters, Ava and Faith, to wait for me, but I didn't think it would take me so long to find this puppy and take her home.' Betsy shrugged.

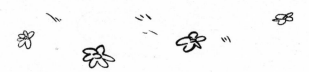

'It seems unfair that we have got lost through no real fault of our own.'

The hare nudged Betsy gently with its wide brown nose.

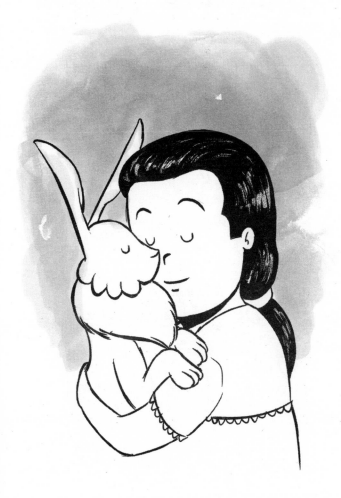

'Sometimes it's hard
to feel grateful
when you're sad,'

the hare agreed.

'But there are
lots of different
ways to make
yourself happy.

I like feeling the warm summer soil under my paws.
Or cold snowflakes dusting the tips of my ears in
winter. And I love the scent of woodland flowers.
I'm grateful for little things like that.'

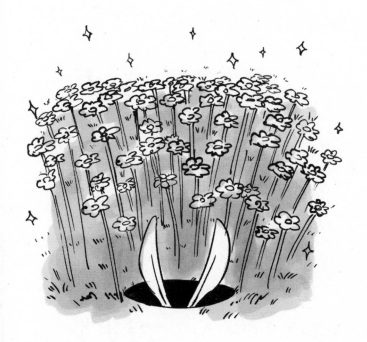

'The butterfly told me the secret is not to worry too much about the past or the future; just be happy for what I have right now.'

'It's not always easy,' admitted the hare, 'but it's always worth searching for the things that lift your heart.

You can find treasure in surprising places.'

Betsy smiled. 'That's true. I wouldn't have found
Clementine if I hadn't crawled through the
scratchy bushes and then the rocky tunnel when I
heard her whimpering.'

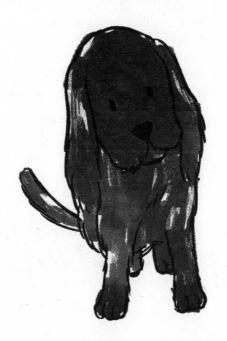

'Exactly!' the hare exclaimed. 'You can be grateful for all the good things that have happened to you precisely *because* you got lost.'

'I wouldn't have met you and the butterfly either,' Betsy beamed. 'You've both been so kind to us.'

'You see? You're already getting the hang of it,' said the hare.

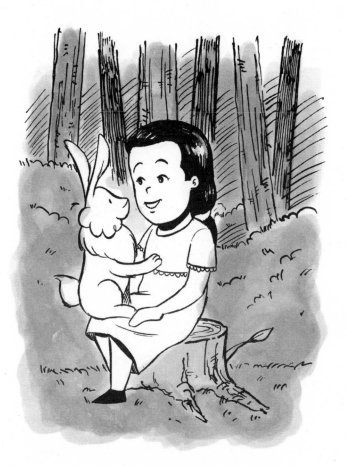

'It's much easier to be kind to people if you're grateful for what you have.'

'But isn't gratitude about being pleased about all the things you own? That's what some grown-ups say.'

The hare sighed. 'No, it's about discovering what

real wealth consists

of _ things like

love and friendship,

caring for others,

not possessions.

Gratitude is what helps us to live a really good life. It's important to remember all the things that we're grateful for. They remind us that life is full of nice things, not just worries.'

'In that case,' said Betsy finally, 'I'm going to make a habit of finding new things to be grateful for every day. That way, it'll be easier to remember just how lucky I am and be happy.'

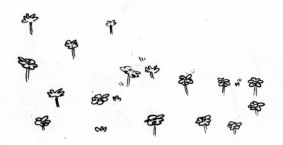

'You can be spandandall too!' Betsy felt the bob and bounce of the hare's enormous back feet, as it started to move away from them across the glade.

'Come on!' the hare called back to them.
'I've got an idea. Follow me!'

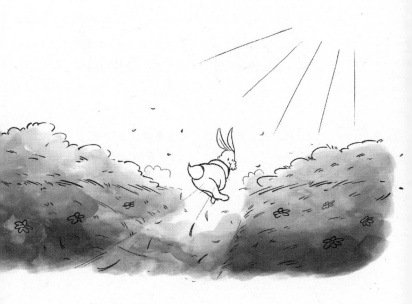

Betsy and Clementine set off eagerly after it, listening out for the sound of the hare's voice and the pounding of its huge feet to orientate themselves,

grateful to be helped by such a kind creature.

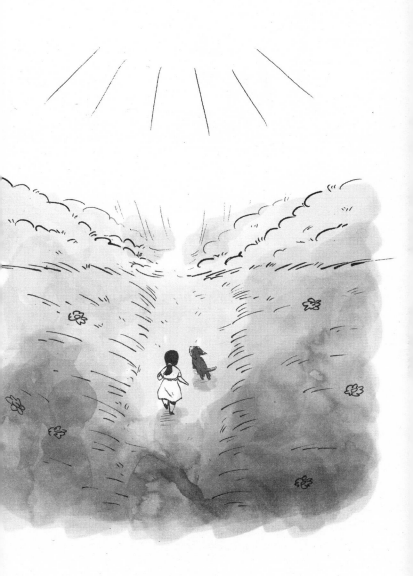

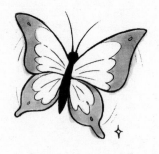

CHAPTER 3

The Impossible is Possible

At the other side
of the glade, the
air filled with loud,
frantic buzzing.

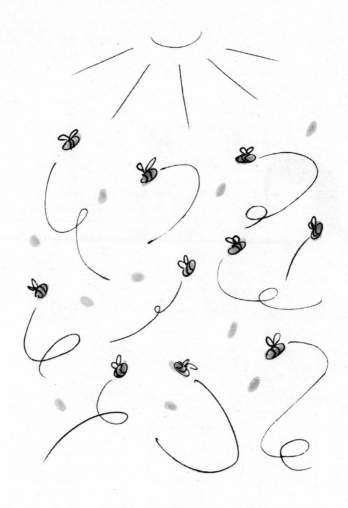

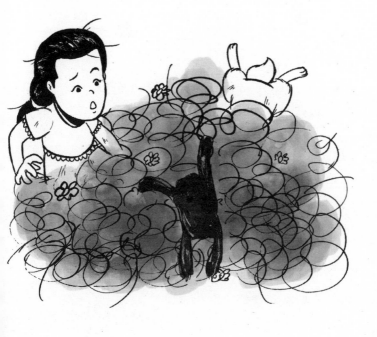

The hare stopped abruptly in its tracks, Clementine crashed into the hare and Betsy tripped over Clementine.

They landed in a tangled heap.

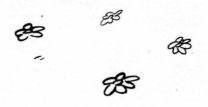

Betsy got up and brushed herself down, while Clementine and the hare shook themselves free of flowers and grass.

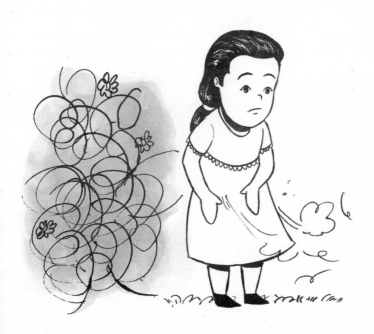

'Whenever you
need to know
anything, always
ask the bees,'

the hare declared. 'They know all there is to know
about the forest, as that's where they like to sip
the flowers. They can tell you everything about the
plants, the flowers, and the trees . . . probably even
the way to the Meadowlands. Their hive is tucked
away in a gnarled old chestnut tree over there.
Can you hear the muffled drone of the worker bees
inside the trunk?'

Betsy could hear a
low monotonous hum
in the distance.

'I can hear something, but aren't bees dangerous?'

The hare didn't respond, but a thump and a swoosh, alongside a faint, 'Goodbye and good luck!' announced its departure into the undergrowth.

The buzzing grew louder. Clementine plonked herself down on her bottom and refused to budge.

Betsy sat down too, trailing her hand through what felt like a carpet of daisies, her fingers lingering over soft petals and furry stalks.

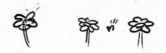

'Please watch where you're sitting!'
a teeny voice buzzed from the
heart of a small flower.

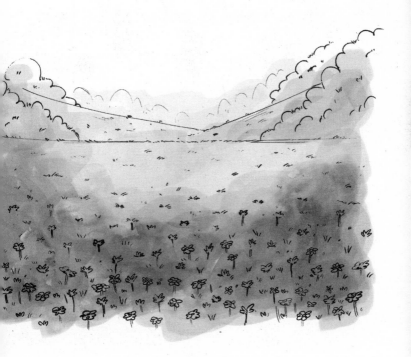

Betsy bent down towards the voice, so close that

she could almost feel
the vibrations of the
bee's tiny wings.

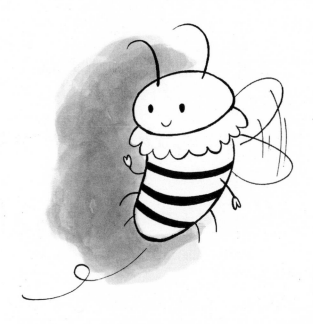

'I think my puppy friend is scared we might be stung
if we go too near to your hive. And, if I'm honest,
I'm a little bit worried too.

Clementine, mind your nose,' she said to the puppy,
who was sniffing noisily at the bee.

'It's easy to get caught up in worrying about the wrong thing,'

said the bee.

'Why would I or any of my friends want to hurt you?'

'I suppose we just thought you might.'
Betsy felt the heat rush to her cheeks.
Why did she think that?

'Did you know you can use your imagination
to make yourself feel happy and curious,
instead of frightened or sad?'

'I hadn't really thought about it.'
Betsy felt slightly dizzy, as she could hear
the bee buzzing in circles around her head.

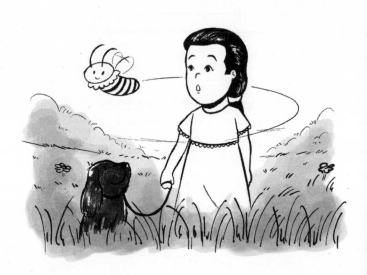

'I know my imagination plays tricks on me sometimes, and I worry about things that aren't really there.'

'If you have any worries like that, you need to tell a friend about them.'

The bee stretched out its wings.
'Or laugh at the idea. Just go, Hah!'

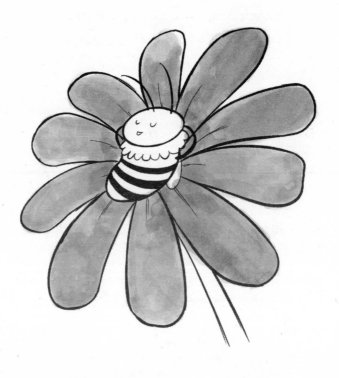

'Hah!'

'There are always ways to use your imagination to make yourself happy. There's no need to be grumpy if you know how to use your imagination well.'

'I'm not grumpy!' Betsy changed the subject. 'But I think Clementine might be quite frightened. She seems to be lost and we're trying to get back to the Meadowlands.'

'Imagination takes courage.'

The bee hummed thoughtfully. 'It means being brave enough to explore new ideas.'

Betsy wondered what sort of new ideas the bee had in mind. 'But what happens then?' she asked.

'When you let your imagination fly, you discover many wonderful things. Just think about bees visiting flowers around the forest and bringing their pollen back to the hive, where it's turned into the most delicious honey.'

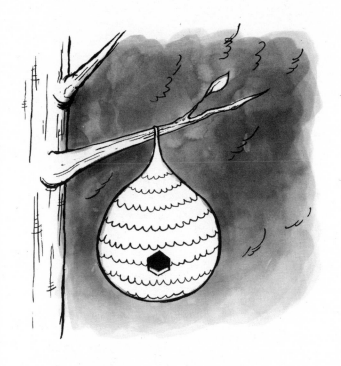

'I do like honey.' Betsy's mouth watered at the thought of sticky, sweet honey smeared all over a piece of fresh bread. Her tummy rumbled. 'And I like making things,' she added.

'Life is all about
making things,'

the bee agreed,

'and doing the
best we can.'

'But what about following the rules? That's what grown-ups say is important.'

'Rules don't always matter when you're being creative. You can create your own world. It all depends on the connections you make with the things you encounter.'

'Oh!' Betsy's face lit up. 'It's a bit like eating cherries – the sudden sweet and sour flavours always makes me think of the start of summer. They're around for such a short time that they're like a doorway into long, warm days and holidays, as well as picnics and playing in the sun all day.'

'It's good to find your own meanings,'

said the bee, 'and to take risks and have adventures.'

'Clementine and I seem to have found ourselves
in the middle of an adventure,' Betsy explained,
'but we would quite like to get back home
before dinnertime.'

'Why not use your imagination to find your way?' suggested the bee.

Clementine tugged on her lead restlessly, reminding Betsy that they needed to keep moving. 'How do we do that?' Betsy asked.

'Well,' said the bee, 'you could start by imagining that you're on the right path. Keep telling yourself: "I'm on my way home". Then visualize your family waiting to greet you with a hug. After all, everybody needs a cuddle, and best of all, it's free. Then let those positive feelings guide you on your way. You'll find your way home in no time. You'll see.'

Betsy patted Clementine on her silky soft head. 'We'll both try,' she promised.

'You know,
sometimes what you
think is impossible,
is actually possible,'

said the bee in a soothing voice.

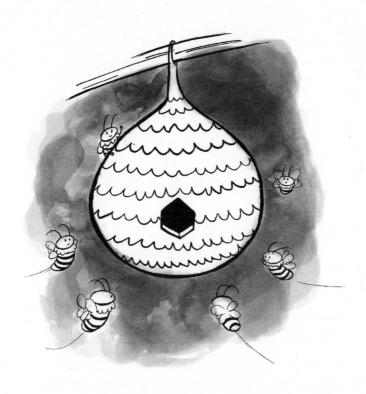

And with that, it said goodbye, then whirred and
murmured, as it meandered lazily across the glade
to join the hive, where the other bees hummed a
noisy welcome.

'We're on our

way home,'

Betsy reassured Clementine. Then she coaxed
Clementine gently around the tree where the bees
had made their hive, pulling softly on the puppy's
lead, muttering encouragement, and listening out for
their buzzing chatter, careful not to get too close and
disturb them.

With a happier heart, Betsy and the puppy went back
into the forest, and this time Clementine seemed
eager to lead the way.

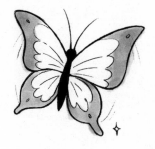

CHAPTER 4

Sing Your Own Song

Twigs snapped loudly beneath their feet. Betsy jumped at the sharp sound. The pounding of her own heart seemed like the loudest thing in the forest.

Clementine was starting to lag a little behind, her tiny feet dawdling behind Betsy, her short legs struggling to keep up.

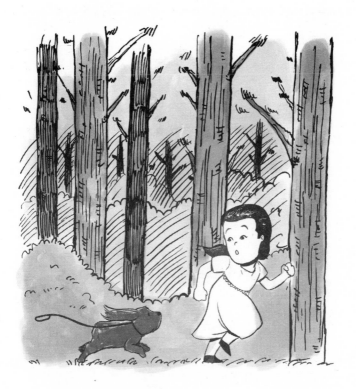

Betsy scooped the puppy into her arms and settled at the foot of a thick tree trunk. The rough bark rubbed against her back.

Betsy could smell pine resin and pollen drifting on the breeze.

'Let's have a rest.'

She closed her eyes briefly as high above them
the song of a bird trilled and twittered.

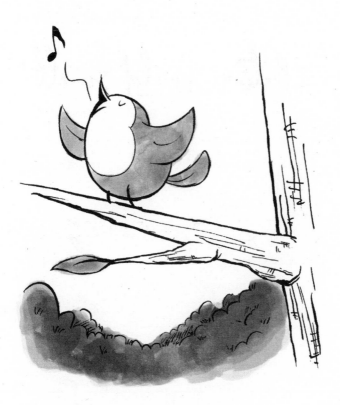

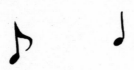

Then a bird in a different tree started to sing too, and then another, and another . . . until the treetops filled with a harmony of birdsong, a joyful sound that wove its way into Betsy's soul.

The music soared and fell, soothing Betsy. And by the time the birds stopped singing, she felt sure everything would be all right.

She started to hum a gentle tune of her own to comfort Clementine, who snuffled and snuggled more closely against her.

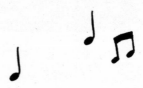

There was a chirp from above. 'I heard you calling.'
A bird tweeted in notes as breezy and bright as a
spring day.

'I was singing to cheer up my puppy,' said Betsy.
'And myself too, I suppose.

Music nearly always
lifts my mood,

and when I get a bit teary or scared,
I sing about how I feel.'

'That's a beautiful song,' said the bird. 'It made me remember how, when I first left the nest, the forest seemed so large and frightening.'

'I liked your song too.' Betsy recalled the comforting sounds floating through the treetops. 'It convinced me and Clementine that things will get better.'

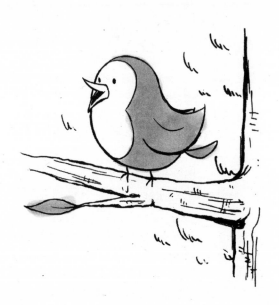

'Music makes the world a happier, better place for everybody.'

The bird flapped its wings noisily. 'It would be a miserable place without it.'

Betsy agreed. 'I'm especially grateful for songbirds like you, because without them there would be no music, and that would be a very sad world indeed.'

'It's almost impossible to imagine a world without tunes and songs.' The bird whistled and warbled high above Betsy's head.

'Music is part of who we are. It's in our very bones and feathers.'

'I don't have feathers.' Betsy ran her hands through her hair, as if to check she was right. 'But I love how music brings everyone together. We all need to sing and dance more often.'

The bird gave a loud trill.

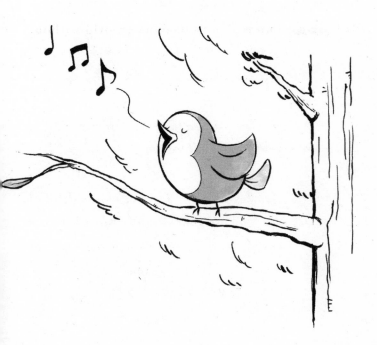

'Songs help us to understand each other and what we are feeling. They help us to understand ourselves too.'

'I wish there was a song that could help me and this little one find our way home.' Betsy tickled Clementine's squidgy, round tummy, sensing the puppy's enjoyment, as Clementine rolled over on to her back so Betsy could rub her tummy more easily.

'Why don't you make one up?' The bird landed on Betsy's shoulder.

'Create a tune that cheers you up and helps you find the courage inside to face whatever is hard for you.'

So, Betsy began to sing. Her voice, clear and strong, floated through the trees, the melody carried high through the branches. The bird joined in, whistling and chirping loudly above their heads.

Clementine jumped up, pulling Betsy to her feet, and they set off together into the forest, stepping in time with renewed energy, to their newfound marching anthem.

Now, the world seemed less confusing and their path felt clearer.

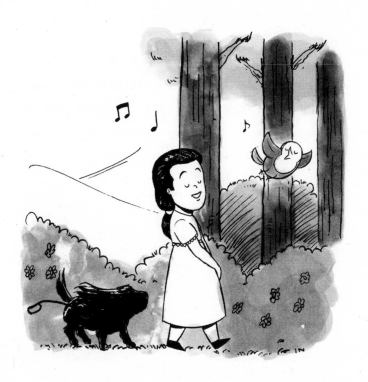

After a while, Betsy realized the bird was no longer accompanying them; no longer flying from tree to tree above them, or enhancing their melody. She and Clementine were on their own again.

Betsy breathed in, and carried on singing her new song, filled with the courage it gave her. And as the notes echoed off the trees surrounding them, creating a rousing chorus of sound that strengthened their hope, they walked and sang of home.

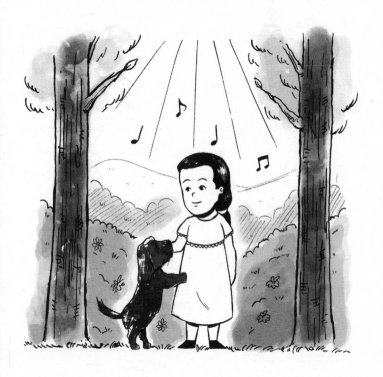

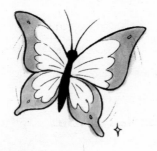

CHAPTER 5

Kindness is a Small Thing

The forest seemed to stretch on and on. Their feet followed a continuous, straight path, never veering to the right or left, apparently without end. Moisture dripped from the trees, large, slow drops landing splat, splat on Betsy's skin.

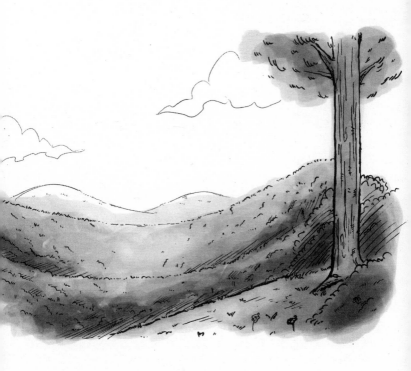

The musty smell
of leaf mould and

ancient vegetation

rose from the

damp ground.

The temperature was dropping and Betsy's stomach rumbled loudly, reminding her that it had been a long time since lunch. The little dog stopped every now and again to drink and splash in dark, cool water that pooled in mossy hollows.

As they passed under a holly tree, with Clementine pulling Betsy slightly to the side to avoid the prickles, they nearly didn't hear the squeak.

'Ow!' said something small.

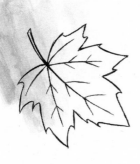

'Who's there? Whatever is the matter?' asked Betsy. She crouched close to the ground, near to where the sound had come from. Her hand grazed a prickly leaf, leaving a faint scratch across her knuckles. She reached out tentatively, sure she was close to a holly bush, and not wanting to fall into it.

'I'm trying to reach the tasty berries,' said the voice. 'But every time I jump up, I hurt myself on the prickles.'

Betsy bent down, and rested her hand on the ground.

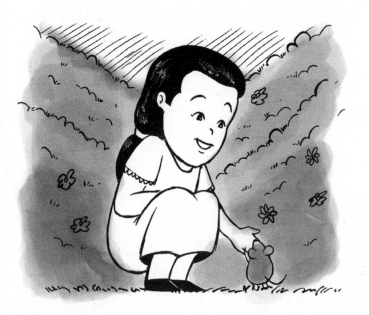

A small, furry creature scurried over her fingers, and she felt a long smooth tail behind tiny, scampering paws.

It was

a mouse.

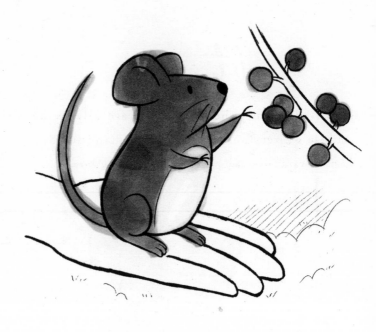

'Let me help you,' Betsy said, as the mouse made himself comfortable on her palm. 'How high do you want to go?' she asked.

She lifted him up, then, listening carefully to the mouse's directions, Betsy held her hand steady when he said he could reach the berries. She waited patiently while he ate. Clementine whined for attention at her feet.

'Delicious!' said the mouse at last. 'Thank you for helping me. That was a very kind thing to do.'

'You're welcome,' said Betsy as she set the mouse down.

'I like being kind. I feel warm inside when I do nice things, and when people are good to each other it creates such a lovely atmosphere.'

'Kindness and helping each other are very important,' replied the mouse. 'But would you mind asking your puppy not to lick me? It's like being washed by a giant pink slug.'

'Clementine, come here!' Betsy pulled the puppy away from the mouse. 'There you go.'

'Thank you.' The mouse dried his face, wiping tiny paws across his nose.

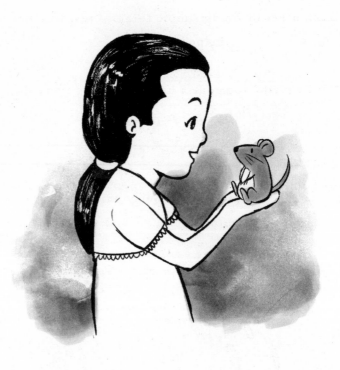

'It's funny, isn't it, how we can make life better for each other by doing simple things – just like you helped me now.

'Or by giving someone a hug and telling them that everything's going to be all right.'

Betsy ran her hands down Clementine's silky ears, letting her know with a gentle touch that everything was okay.

'Everything is going to be all right.'

The mouse scampered onto Betsy's shoulder.

'Thank you.' Betsy laughed as the mouse's whiskers tickled her. 'Clementine and I both needed to hear that. I'm not sure if we're heading the right way for home. I'm doing my best to be brave and cheerful for Clementine, but it's getting harder,' she said. She paused for a moment, then continued.

'Sometimes I have to remind myself that I can choose not to be sad or grumpy. That makes life better for me and for everyone else. By having positive thoughts, I imagine how I can help others too, and then I immediately feel better.'

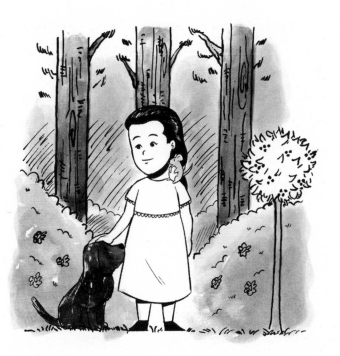

'Kindness is all about making the right choices, isn't it? We can always choose to be kind and it's very easy to do.' The mouse pushed his nose softly into Betsy's neck.

'Kindness can also just mean doing something small every day that makes a big difference,' Betsy said as she reached out slowly to avoid the prickly holly leaves and used her fingers to locate some more juicy holly berries for the mouse. Then she pulled them off one by one, taking care to avoid being scratched. She handed them to him.

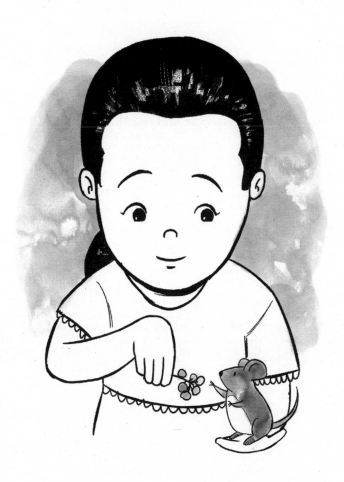

'The more people do good things, the more the world could be a really happy place.'

The mouse accepted the berries with a gentle nuzzle to Betsy's hand. 'If we treat each other kindly then we'll all get along.'

Betsy paused, her eyes flickering from left to right, her lips pursed in concentration. 'I've thought about kindness a lot,' she said eventually, 'and I am sure that it's good for you.

Kindness makes you live longer, because if you do kind things for others it makes you feel really good about yourself.

'We can choose to be kind to ourselves as well,' said the mouse, although it was difficult to hear what he said as he chomped on a holly berry, the juice dribbling off his nose.

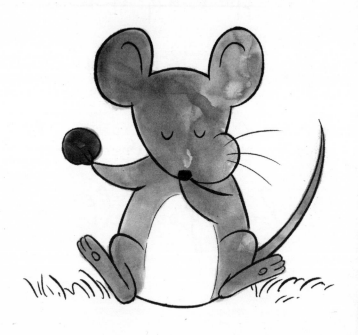

'That's true,' said Betsy. 'We need to look after ourselves because

we only get one body and one life,

so it's important to make sure that we get the best out of them both.'

The mouse offered Betsy his last berry and held it
out till it tickled her arm. 'Would you like one?'

'Thank you, but we'd better not. Holly berries aren't
good for me or Clementine.'

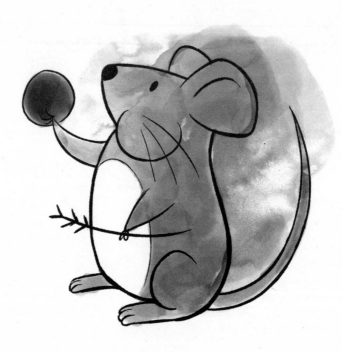

'Then what would you like to eat?' asked the mouse.

'Clementine would like a long cool drink of water,' said Betsy, 'and I would love a big slice of apple pie.'

'I don't have any pie, but I do know where there are some hazelnuts. Would you like me to take you there?'

'Yes, please,' said Betsy.

'Whenever someone's kind to me,
I try to be kind in return. Come.'

The mouse climbed onto Clementine's back and tugged gently on the dog's lead, directing her left and right, until they finally arrived at a stream. Water burbled noisily over smooth pebbles, gurgling as it trickled along its course. 'The water is lovely and fresh here,' the mouse said. Clementine's tongue lapped at the water, then she shook her head, splashing water over Betsy's legs.

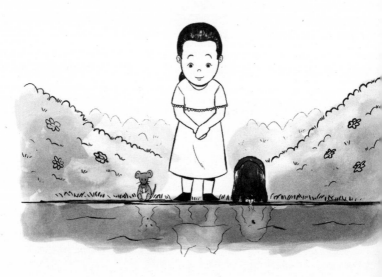

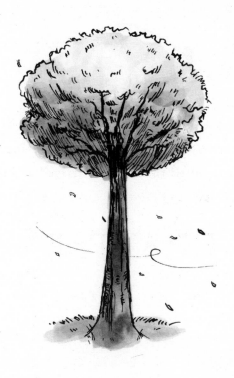

'You will find ripe hazelnuts to eat too,'
said the mouse. 'Stretch out your hands.
They're on the trees to both your left and right.'

With that, he said goodbye and scurried away.

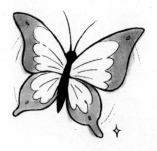

CHAPTER 6

Face Your Fears

The breeze blew gently, fluttering Betsy's hair. Leaves whispered in the distance. Clementine drank deeply from the stream, then barked excitedly.

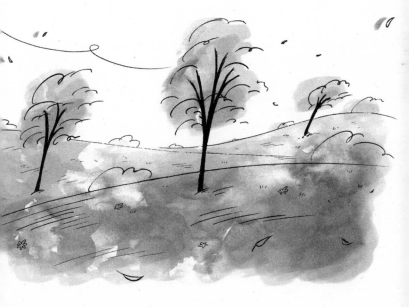

With a tug at her lead, the puppy pulled Betsy off to the right. Then she stopped, her paws scratching against a nearby tree trunk, barking at something above them.

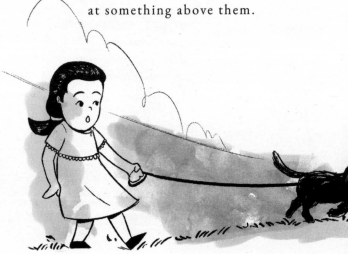

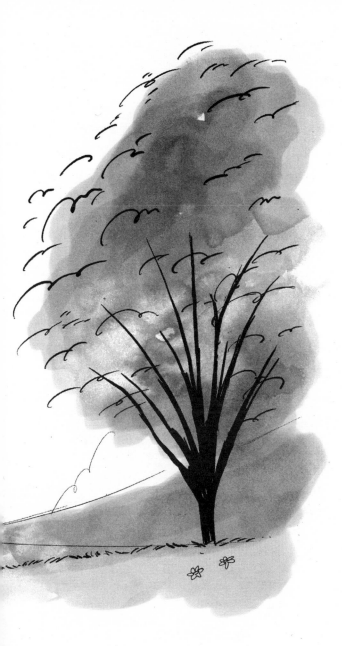

Betsy felt as if she was treading on pebbles. The soles of her feet sensed hard, sharp shells beneath her shoes. The mouse had mentioned hazelnut trees, and the ground crunched as she moved forwards. She reached down and touched the ground with her hand. Sure enough, cracked nutshells littered the earth.

Betsy searched beneath the tree and ran her hands up its smooth, solid trunk and through its lowest branches. But she found no nuts. She grabbed the next branch she came across and gave it a light shake.

Something round and hard dropped on her head.

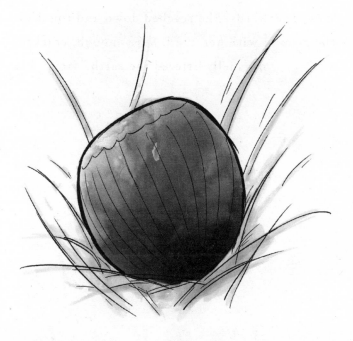

'Ouch!' she exclaimed, as a smooth, hard-cased
hazelnut landed at her feet.

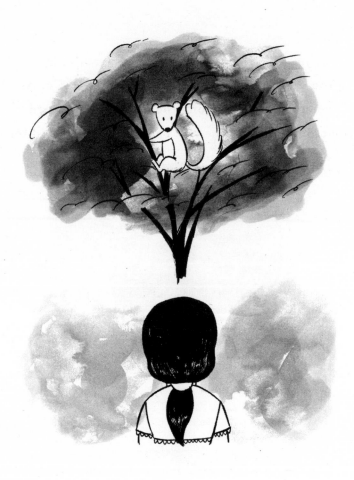

Something chattered and squealed above her. 'You can have that one if you like,' called a cross voice from high among the leaves. Betsy heard something move in the tree overhead, a tail brushing the leaves as a creature moved through the foliage, its claws scraping the bark, as it scampered along the branches on light feet.

'What are you doing up there?' asked Betsy.

'Gathering nuts and getting ready for winter,' came the voice again, from far off the ground.

A squirrel then, Betsy thought. 'Aren't you afraid to climb all the way up there?' She craned her neck in the direction of the animal.

'I have to be a little bit brave every day,'

the squirrel shouted from up high. 'Sometimes we all have to do things we might not want to do, but

we need to face our fears and do them anyway,

even when it's hard.'

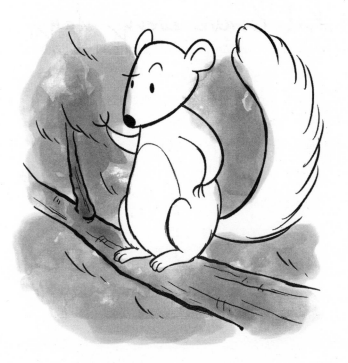

'I'm very hungry,' said Betsy, as her stomach gurgled loudly, 'but I can't risk climbing up the tree. If I fall, who will take Clementine home?'

'Yes, but the hazelnuts can't climb down to you,' the squirrel said cheekily, and threw another nut down at Betsy's feet.

'I'll find a way,'

said Betsy.

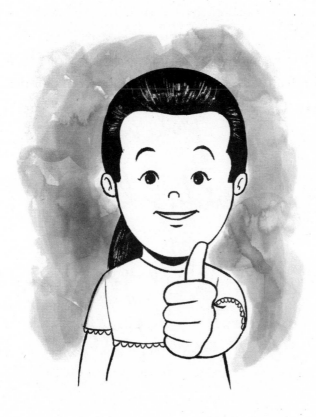

'Whenever I'm upset that I can't do something, because it wouldn't be safe or easy, I think of how I might be able to fix that.

I put my shoulders back and tell myself, "You can do this!"

When the world feels positive, then the world is positive.' The squirrel's voice was kinder this time.

Betsy turned to Clementine, who had now stopped barking. 'Come on, my lovely puppy dog, find me a long stick!'

Clementine jumped up, wanting to play. Sticks were one of her favourite things. The soft, velvety pads of her paws patted Betsy's legs. Where was the stick? She looked at Betsy's empty hands, but then seemed to understand what Betsy wanted.

Betsy heard scrabbling about in the bushes behind her, a loud rustle of dry leaves, then a scraping noise as something was dragged over the crunchy nutshells. A moment later, Clementine plonked a large stick across Betsy's toes.

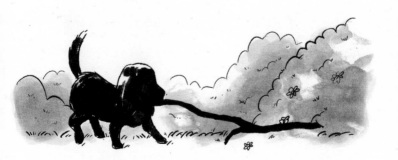

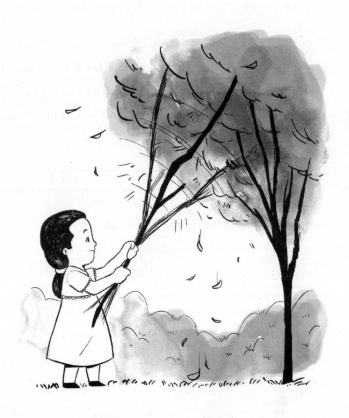

Clementine tugged at the stick when Betsy went to grab it. Playtime! she thought. She let Betsy take it from her. 'Good girl.' Betsy patted her head.

She took the stick in one hand and reached up as high as she could, waving the stick above her head, trying to rattle the branches and knock down some nuts. She knew there were some on the tree, hanging like delicious treasure hidden among the leaves.

Little bits of the tree rained down around her, becoming tangled and knotted in her hair. Betsy sneezed, as a leaf landed on her nose. But, although she felt the impact of twigs and debris on her head, there were no satisfying crashes to indicate that any hazelnuts had fallen too.

'Ow! This is actually very difficult!' she said, when she accidentally hit herself with the stick for the third time.

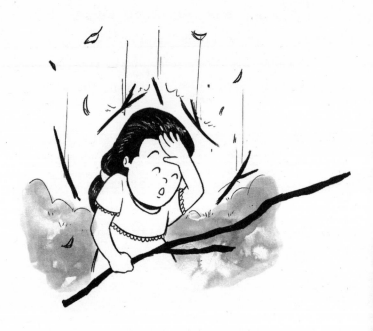

The squirrel called down,

'If you get upset,
it's all right to
have a little cry.

But take a few deep breaths and you'll find that you
feel better and are ready to start again.'

'Sometimes,' muttered Betsy – although whether she was talking to the squirrel or herself, she didn't really know – 'I find it hard to control my emotions. They can take over. But surely you can imagine how this is making me feel?' Her stomach growled, to emphasize her point.

'If you're worried or upset about something, then let that worry out and talk to someone about it.'

The squirrel sounded closer now.

'You're never too old to ask for help.'

Betsy dropped the stick and crossed her arms in frustration. She'd had enough and was close to giving up.

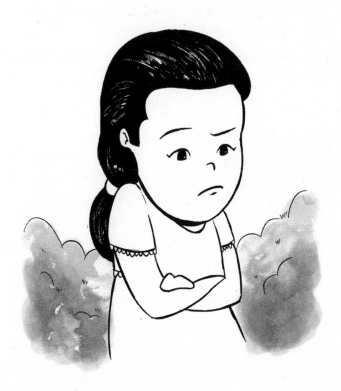

'You're nearly there,' said the squirrel encouragingly.

After a moment's consideration, Betsy took a few deep breaths, picked up the stick and headed back to the tree.

She held the stick at one end, making it as long as it could be, then stood on tiptoe and poked the stick into the branches again. She moved it from side to side, hearing it swish through the leaves. Nothing happened.

She tried again,

sweeping the stick in a wider arc through the branches. Thunk! A large cluster of nuts fell to the ground.

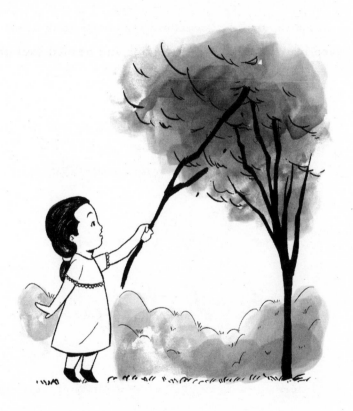

'Here, these are yours,' said the squirrel, appearing suddenly at her side, its bushy tail sweeping along her arm. It tipped the nuts into her waiting hands. 'It was very brave of you to keep on going.'

'In order to survive, we have to carry on, don't we?'

said Betsy, as she searched for a stone to crack open the nutshells.

She shared the hazelnuts with the squirrel, who opened one with a crunch and started to nibble away.

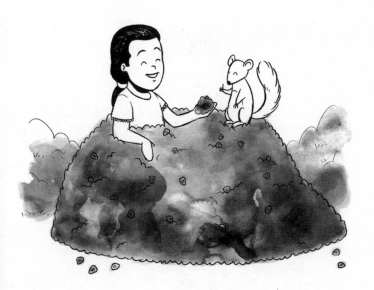

'I'm sorry you can't eat these nuts too, but I'll get you home soon for your dinner,' Betsy promised Clementine. 'Everything I've learned helps to keep me healthy and positive, and I am going to look after you too.'

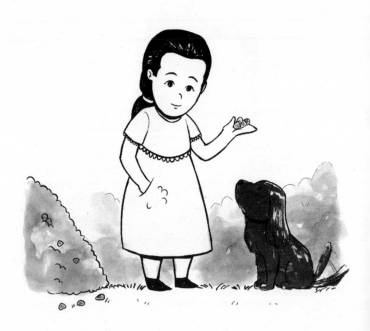

'That's better.' The squirrel stretched happily.
'I'm not hungry now.'

Betsy popped a couple of nuts in her pocket,
to save for later.

'It's important not
to give up, even
when you feel lost.'

'And are you lost?' asked the squirrel.

'Yes, and we want to get back safely to the Meadowlands before nightfall.' She knew the day was nearly over.

Cool air tickled her face and the sun no longer warmed her skin with the same intensity as before.

The ground felt slightly damp and cold
around her feet.

'I know a path out of the woods,' said the
squirrel, 'but it winds through the most dangerous
part of the forest.'

Betsy didn't hesitate. 'Let's go!' she said.
'Facing our fears is the only way forward.'

And holding on tightly to Clementine's lead, she and her trusting puppy followed the squirrel along the trail, following the sensation of its bouncing feet, as the bushy-tailed creature bounded ahead as though its little feet were on springs.

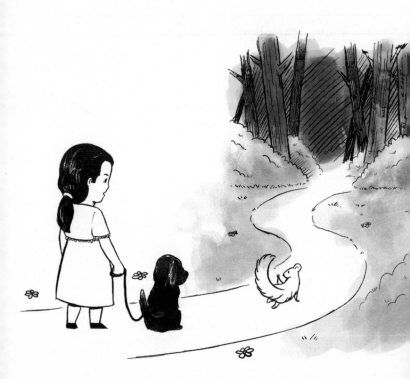

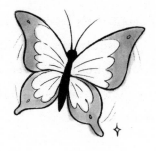

CHAPTER 7

You Can Only Be Brave When Scared

They travelled along a smooth, winding path for a while, until the squirrel stopped.

'This is the right way,' he said, 'but I have to leave you here. Just stay on this path and you should find your way. Farewell and good luck.'

Betsy and Clementine pressed on.

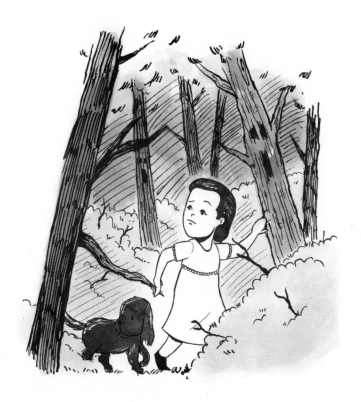

The trees and bushes moved closer, overhanging the path. They seemed to grab at them from all around, their branches and roots creating obstacles and hurdles in their way. Betsy's feet scuffed against exposed tree stumps and tripped over protruding rocks, as she staggered over uneven ground. She stumbled, trying not to fall, feeling her way cautiously. Every now and then Clementine stopped, as if she was listening or searching for something in their surroundings.

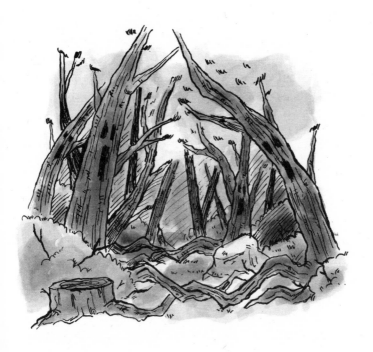

The forest became ever more silent and still, the air thick with moisture.

Water droplets dripped from above and splashed off Betsy's hands. Sometimes, a branch snapped or something rustled overhead, as if they were being followed. Was something watching them?

Betsy stopped for a rest. At her feet, she felt Clementine tremble, as she flopped to the ground, her head on her paws. The little dog was exhausted and her little legs were struggling to continue.

'You've helped me get this far,' Betsy said to Clementine, who she could hear panting by her side. 'Let me carry you now.' She picked up the small puppy and cuddled her tightly, whispering words of comfort into her silky ear.

We must be nearly there. Not far to go.

'And when we get back,' Betsy promised, 'I'll help you find your family. But I do hope we can stay friends for ever. We make a good team, don't we – with me looking after you and you looking after me? We can be best friends.'

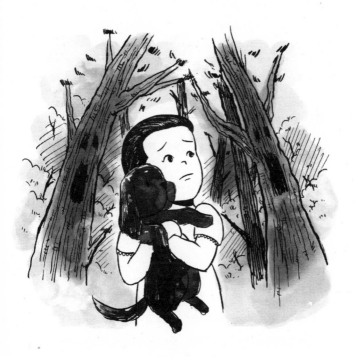

not a sound could be heard, as if all noise had been swallowed up by the forest.

Brambles ripped at Betsy's legs, rocks nearly tripped her up, yet on she went, deeper into the forest, following the squirrel's path, with Clementine clutched tightly in her arms, glad that she wasn't on her own.

The further they went, the more the trees seemed like creatures leaning in, claws out, so close that their branches seemed to grab at her and scratch her arms. Betsy pushed them away, worried that at some point, something else – something more dangerous – might actually grab hold of her. The day started to fade, the light perfume of leaves and grass replaced by the heavy, musty smell of mushrooms and forgotten secrets.

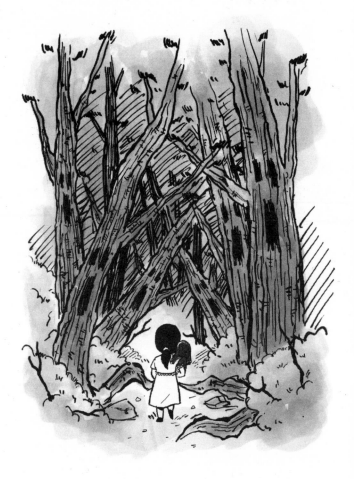

Betsy sensed the
darkness, as it
fell like a deep,
heavy blanket
over the wood,
muffling everything
in its path.

Her steps slowed.

She held one hand out in front of her face, waving it gently in the space ahead, to stop from bumping into a tree and hurting herself. As she walked, Betsy listened to the forest, alert for any sound, any scratch or rustle nearby that might tell her where they were, or let her know they weren't alone. But it was eerily silent. The cloying smells of damp mushrooms were alien and claustrophobic. The twigs and branches sharp and hostile, almost defensive against her outstretched fingers. She trembled, trying to be brave.

'It's all right to feel afraid,'

she whispered to Clementine, hoping she sounded more confident than she felt.

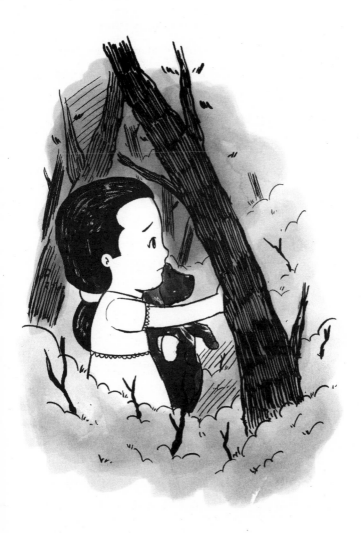

'We all have different emotions, and fears, and worries, and there is nothing wrong with experiencing any of them.

'Some fears are even good,'

she said, as calmly as she could, her heart thumping behind her ribs. 'Like being scared of a lion. Because if you weren't afraid, you might climb into the lions' enclosure at the zoo. And that probably wouldn't end well, would it?'

A loud crash shattered her train of thought. Betsy jumped, startled by the sudden noise.

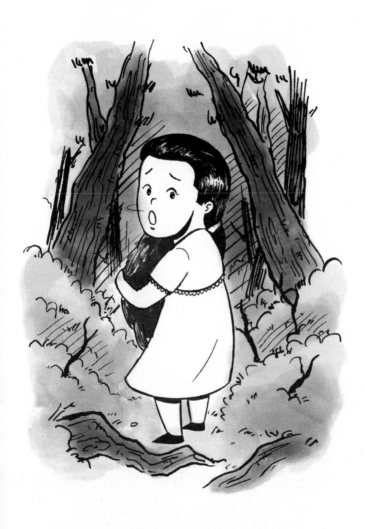

'Who's there?' she cried, clutching the puppy
even tighter.

'Only me,' said a friendly voice near her knees. Betsy smelled dusty tunnels with a hint of succulent berries. She reached down and ran a tentative hand over a bristly coat, short legs, and a long nose, then exhaled in relief. A badger.

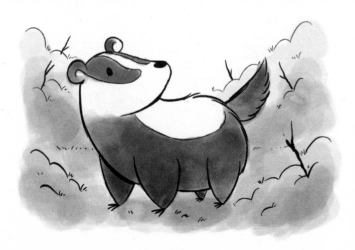

'You frightened us!' said Betsy. 'We thought you were a lion!'

'Sorry about that,' said the badger. 'I was enjoying an evening stroll, but tripped over a twig.'

'Aren't you scared of being alone here? I'm sure it's getting dark now,' Betsy said. 'The wood feels like it's gone to sleep.'

'The dark is a natural thing.' the badger replied.

'The stars come out and light up the sky, and there's really nothing to be frightened about.

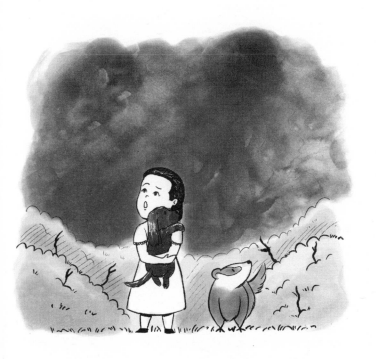

And on starless nights, nothing is really any different
— it just seems that way if you're not used to it.'

The puppy squirmed and whimpered in Betsy's arms.
'That's easy for you to say,' Betsy said, and she kissed
Clementine on the top of her head. 'You're used to
being out at night and know your way around.'

'True,' said the badger.

'It's all right to be scared by things, but there are some fears that you should get rid of, as they can get in the way.

And one of those is definitely being scared of the dark. It can make you less able to do what you want to do . . . whatever that is.'

'We want to follow this path to the edge of the forest,' said Betsy, 'and find our way home, but we keep tripping up, losing our way, and are not sure we are actually heading for the Meadowlands.'

The badger looked up. Betsy's mouth was fixed in a determined line, as she stroked Clementine, trying to hide her own fear from the puppy.

'In that case, come with me. I can help.'

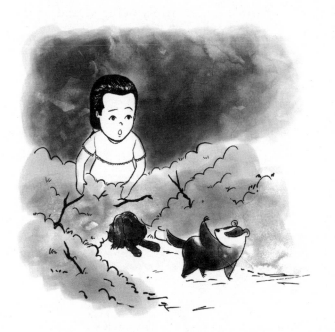

Betsy set Clementine down and placed a hand on the
badger's bristly back. The girl, the puppy, and the
badger walked in companionable silence for a while,
with Betsy and Clementine taking comfort from the
steady presence of the badger, until

Betsy realized
that she didn't feel
scared at all.

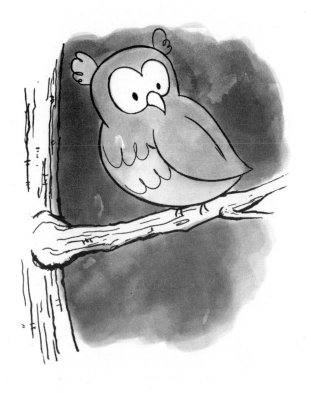

An owl hooted, a soft, resonant tone, welcoming the approaching night. Betsy felt more space around her, as the air thinned and the trees eased back from the path. A few gentle branches tickled her hair, no longer grabbing at them or impeding their way.

The path became firmer and more regular underfoot, as if it were well-trodden. Wood smoke drifted on the breeze, a reminder of home.

'Sometimes,' said the badger, as if he had been busy thinking,

'you just have to reach out, and then you find that everything is all right.'

'We can really only be brave when we're scared.' Betsy recalled her pounding heartbeat and their difficult journey through the woods. 'There are times when we just have to keep on trying.

That's all we can do in the end — try our best.'

Betsy felt the badger come to a halt. She reached down and felt grass around her ankles.

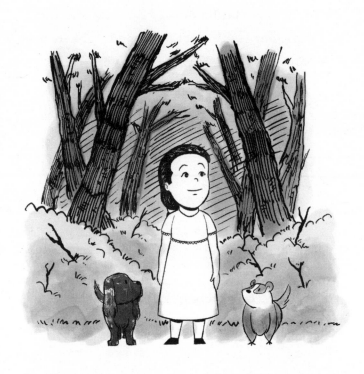

'Here,' he said. 'This is where the forest ends.'

'I wish I could show you how grateful I am to you for leading us here.

Sometimes a hug is all I can offer by way of thanks.

So, thank you.' Betsy hugged the badger hard.

The badger squeezed her back. 'Now we both feel much better.' He laughed.

'Will you say goodbye to all the animals that we met in the woods?' Betsy asked. 'They were so helpful – even the squirrel, who teased me at first.'

'There's no need to say goodbye to them,' said the badger. 'After all, you still carry them in your heart.'

Ahead, the meadow grasses sighed and shivered in the breeze. And then, coming closer and closer,

Betsy heard familiar voices calling her name:

her sisters, Ava and Faith, and her parents calling for her loudly.

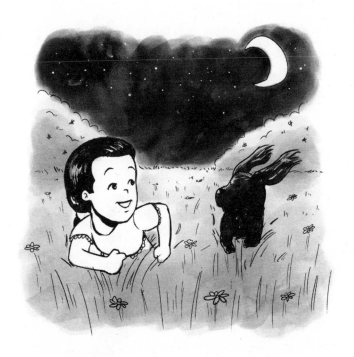

'There she is!' cried Ava.

Betsy was swept up in their embrace. She breathed in the comforting smell of her mother's hair and felt the strength of her father's arms and her sisters' relief as they all cuddled her tightly. It seemed the bee's promise had come true – the impossible had become possible; they had found their way home.

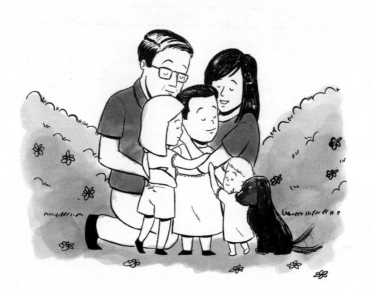

'Ava told us what happened and we've been searching for you everywhere.' Her mother's relief escaped in a laugh that sounded almost like a sob.

'And who's this?' her father asked. Clementine peered out shyly from behind Betsy's legs, and reached over to take a closer look at baby Faith. There was a slurp and Faith giggled as Clementine licked her.

'This is Clementine. She was lost in the woods, but I found her and brought her home. Please can we keep her?' asked Betsy.

'Oh, yes please,' said Ava and Faith together, already smitten by Clementine's silky fur and happy snuffles.

'I think I know where Clementine comes from,' said their mother.

Betsy's heart sank. Clementine already had somewhere to go to.

But then she heard her mother say, 'There's a farm nearby with a sign that says they have a litter of puppies who need good homes.'

'Well, it looks like Clementine's already found one,' said their father. 'I'll go and speak to the farmer while you all go back to the house. Betsy and Clementine must be very hungry and it's nearly bedtime.'

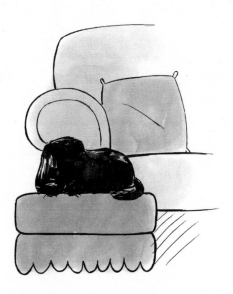

Surrounded by the love of her family,

Betsy knew that
she and Clementine
were truly home and
out of the woods.

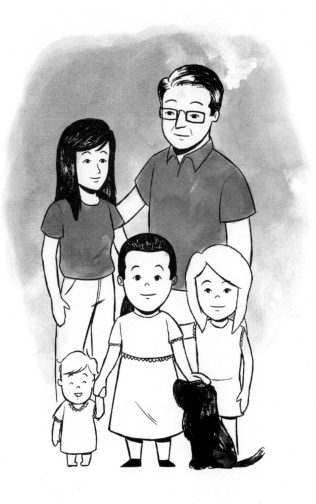

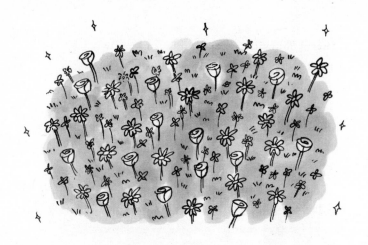

ACKNOWLEDGEMENTS

I never thought that something this amazing would happen to me – I have my own published book! There have been many people who have been very helpful, considerate and full of generosity along the way that I would like to thank.

The journey to this book all started when I was 6, and I had the idea of making a YouTube channel called Betsy's Positive Videos, which was created during the first lockdown. During this time, I also wrote my first attempt at a book about a parrot that eats a burger! My kind braille tutor Keren helped me produce this, including swelled pictures. I really wanted it to go on sale at my local bookshop, Chorleywood Bookshop, and Sheryl (the owner) accepted my unpublished book. Then the journey began with so many people being part of this story:

Sheryl Shurville – thank you for not only putting my book on the shelf but also putting us in contact with Wendy Holden. You went above and beyond for me.

Wendy Holden – thank you for helping us by giving us so much of your time and wanting the very best for me. Thanks also for putting us in touch with Bev.

Bev James – thank you *so* much, Bev, for not only being a wonderful agent but for sending me lovely voice messages and treats. Without you, this book wouldn't be here. We think your words come from your heart that's made of gold and I love your accent.

Sue Belfrage – when we first met, we had a good old joke about my cuddly toys. I think we all agree that you have a spandandall sense of humour and you were just perfect for helping me with my book – thank you.

Lisa Milton and the HarperCollins team – thank you for being so excited about my book, always listening and for all the fantastic ideas.

Emanuel Santos – thank you for your amazing drawings. Even though I cannot see the pictures, just knowing that they are there, adding something to the story and that it looks like me, means a lot to me.

Fearne Cotton – thank you for sending me lovely messages and spreading the love for my positive videos. I am so pleased you have done the foreword and audio for my book. Thank you for featuring me in your book too!

RNIB – thank you so much for being a fantastic charity and adapting my book into braille so that I and other braille readers can enjoy it.

To Mummy and Daddy – thank you for being such outstanding role models to me and supporting me with my book. I love both your wonderful sense of humours.

To my sisters, Ava and Faith – thank you for being my cheeky little sisters. Despite all the arguments, I hope you know I will always love you, and I know you will always love me.

Nanny and Grandad – thank you for keeping the secret of my book, having us over for sleepovers, for all the treats, but most of all for always being there for me.

All my wider family and friends – thank you for always helping me, and fundraising for charities close to my heart. You've helped me through operations, treatments, or just simply cheered me on. Thank you for helping me live life to the full!

Staff and friends at Chorleywood Primary School – Thanks for your guidance, kindness and generosity. Special shout-out to my learning support, Mrs Marandola, who has always been there for me. She has taken the time to learn Braille, for which my family and I are so grateful.

Keren Hedges – for making wonderful resources, teaching me at 7.15 a.m. in the morning Monday–Friday, and being so committed to what she does.

Watford General Hospital – for supporting me through chemotherapy and giving me the opportunity to be on *Gareth Malone's Christmas Concert* which I loved! Special shout-out to Vasanta Nanduri for being at the end of the phone day or night.

Great Ormond Street Hospital – for helping me treat my brain tumour and always being upbeat, nurturing and hardworking.

To all you readers – thank you for taking the time to read my book; I really appreciate it and I hope you enjoy it.

Tori Youens, Tracey Hunter and Melissa Cox from Hertfordshire Vision Impairment Team – you are amazingly positive and kind people who always want the best for me and know how to help me.

Rennie Grove Hospice – special mention to Jane from the Pepper Nursing Team who regularly visits me and puts up with my crazy ideas.

HQ
An imprint of HarperCollins*Publishers* Ltd
1 London Bridge Street
London SE1 9GF

www.harpercollins.co.uk

HarperCollins*Publishers*
Macken House, 39/40 Mayor Street Upper,
Dublin 1, D01 C9W8, Ireland

This edition 2023

10 9 8 7 6 5 4 3 2 1

First published in Great Britain by HQ, an imprint of HarperCollins*Publishers* Ltd 2022

Text Copyright © Betsy Griffin 2022

Illustrations © HarperCollins Publishers 2022

Betsy Griffin asserts the moral right to be identified as the author of this work.
A catalogue record for this book is available from the British Library.

ISBN 978-0-00-851964-3

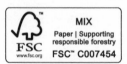

This book is produced from independently certified FSC™ paper to ensure responsible
forest management.

For more information visit: www.harpercollins.co.uk/green

Design & Art Direction: Emily Voller
Illustrator: Emanuel Santos

Printed and bound in the UK using 100% renewable electricity at CPI Group (UK) Ltd